GLUTEN FREE FOOD AHEAD,
On the road to Gluten Free Cooking!

By

Daren P. Solomon

Table of Contents

NOTES:

PREFACE

Growing up in a small New England town as part of a large family I saw firsthand what fun and hard work it is to prepare a great meal. The whole family participated in the cooking, whether it was a quick meal on a school night or Sunday Dinner when friends and family would stop by. Often the extra seats at the table would number more than a dozen.

When I was eighteen I moved out of the house and into my first apartment. My parents gave me a copy of "The Joy of Cooking" and a plastic box filled with index cards of our family recipes. Over the years I cooked my way through the book and cards, calling my parents occasionally to ask advice. In that time I've perfected many of those recipes I inherited, added modern twists occasionally and even created a few new cards of my own to add to the family trove.

Most of us find out about Celiac Disease after suffering chronic stomach pains for years. When our daughter was three years old we were at our wits end trying to figure out why she always had stomach pain. Finally her doctor suggested we test her for gluten allergies. The test came back positive and we immersed ourselves in researching all we could find about gluten free foods. Along the way our whole family got tested and mine came back positive as well.

Though relieved we identified the problem, the challenge we faced was finding a new way to buy and cook our favorite dishes. When we were first diagnosed I began calling it the "$5 Disease" because it seemed everything from a loaf of bread to crackers and pasta all cost $5. Sometimes three times what the wheat version costs! The Gluten Free choices were either nonexistent or what was available was bland and unsatisfying. It was very frustrating, especially when we went out to eat.

At the time we owned three Pizza restaurants and I thought "I can do better than this on my own!" So I went back to my trusty recipe cards and began working on alternatives to substitute other flours for wheat. Some recipes were easy to convert while others took a bit longer. I've often said that "baking is an art." I have found this to be especially true for Gluten Free baking. My first breads were absolute failures. They rose so perfectly in the oven only to collapse while cooling over and over again! The French Baguette recipe you'll find in the following pages took me six years to develop and is one of my favorites.

The recipes in this book are intended for busy parents who are looking for easy to prepare gluten free foods that they and their children can enjoy. I've included "Tips" for those with less experience in a kitchen. My hope is that after reading this book you will have a quick and delicious Gluten Free response when your child comes into the kitchen and says "*I'm starving, what's for dinner?*"

Bon Apetit

Daren

TIPS & TECHNIQUES

If you are new to the kitchen or rarely cook, below are some quick and easy tips that every cook should know or learn in order to improve their techniques and enhance their finished work:

What the heck is Mise en Place???

In a commercial kitchen or restaurant the "Mise" as it is known, simply means having all the ingredients and cooking utensils within an arm's reach. It is imperative to be organized in order to cook a properly prepared dish without frustration or stress. Step One of the Mise is **READ** through the recipe and gather your ingredients, utensils and dishes <u>entirely</u> before you begin cooking.

Always be sure to CONTROL YOUR HEAT!!

More meals are ruined or stressed over because the cook does not adjust the heat appropriately. There are times you'll want to cook on high heat. However, most recipes require a steady medium heat with momentary increase in the heat or a reduced heat to simmer during the cooking process.

How to make a Roux:

In a saucepan Melt two (2) Tablespoons of Butter over medium high heat. Add three (3) Tablespoons of Gluten Free Flour (All Purpose or White Rice Flour work best for most sauces). Whisk briskly to blend together. Lower the heat to medium and continue stirring. Slowly begin to add the liquid (usually cream or pan drippings) stirring constantly. Add the Roux to the dish when ready.

How and why to make a *Mirepoix?*

A Mirepoix is blend of Carrot, Onion and Celery. The vegetables are diced or roughly chopped with quantities determined by each recipe. The Mirepoix is typically sauteed. There are many recipes that call for a Mirepoix either by name or by ingredient. It's often used in soups, sauces, roasted dishes and braising meats just to name a few.

How to make **Herb Butter:**

There are many varieties of Herb Butter and so many dishes that pair well with it that everyone should have one or two they can reliably count on. A basic Garlic-Herb Butter consists of one (1) stick of Butter, three (3) Tablespoons of Herbs (ie. Oregano, Basil & Tarragon), one (1) clove of Fresh Garlic hand-mixed together in a bowl. Add a pinch of Salt & Pepper to taste. Lay a piece of plastic film on the counter and spoon the Butter in the center. Roll the plastic film creating a cylinder shape and refrigerate. It will keep for about a week in the refrigerator or a few months in the freezer.

How to **Clarify Butter:**

Cut the Butter into small pieces and place in a small sauce pan over medium heat. Bring to a boil. Reduce heat to medium-low for just about a minute to let any excess water evaporate. Remove from heat and let cool for two (2) minutes. Skim the foamy top with a spoon and discard. Pour just the liquid into measuring cup or bowl for immediate use. Leave white solids in sauce pan.

How to **Roast Garlic:**

Loosely wrap the head of Garlic (still in it's skin) in aluminum foil. Place in a preheated oven at 350 degrees. Roast for 30-40 minutes. Remove from the oven, unwrap the foil to let the Garlic cool. When ready to use, cut the Garlic in half and squeeze the cloves from each half. Refrigerate for later use. It should keep in the refrigerator for about a week.

How to **Separate Eggs:**

Place two (2) bowls on the counter. Crack one Egg over the first bowl passing the Yolk back and forth between the two halves of the shells letting the Egg White drip into the bowl. Pour Yolk into second bowl. Discard shell and repeat with remaining Eggs. Put any unused Egg Whites or Yolks in a sealed container and keep refrigerated for use at a later time.

How to *Hard-Boil Eggs*:

Gently place the Eggs in a 4 quart pot and cover with cold water with a pinch of salt. Turn the heat to medium-high and cover with a lid. When the water comes to a boil turn off the heat, but leave the lid on for 15 minutes. Place the Eggs in a bowl of ice water for approximately five (5) minutes to stop the cooking process. Once cooled, peel the eggs and rinse any bits of shell off.

How to *Poach an Egg:*

In a saucepan bring water almost to a boil. Pour in 2 Tablespoons of Vinegar. Stir the water to create a swirling motion. Crack an Egg(s) into a small dish and gently release into the swirling water. Shut off the heat. Remove Egg(s) from the water after five (5) minutes and use immediately.

How to <u>*KNEAD*</u> *Gluten Free Dough:*

Some Dough (like Banana Bread) will form a batter in the mixing bowl and will remain loose in the pan. Other Dough (like 3-2-1 Pie Dough) will require kneading by hand. To knead, use this simple method: Sprinkle Flour on the work surface. Turn the Dough out onto the Flour. Dust the top of the Dough and begin pressing down and forward. Fold all the Dough back to the middle. Press down and forward again. Fold back to the middle and repeat. Sprinkle more Flour if the Dough remains sticky. Continue until it becomes elastic and pliable.

How to easily <u>*ROLL*</u> *Gluten Free Dough:*

Grease a sheet of parchment paper. Turn out Dough onto the greased paper. Grease another sheet of parchment paper and lay the greased side down over the Dough. Begin rolling in all directions. Lift the top paper and fold all the Dough back to the middle. Grease the top paper again (only if necessary) and lay back down. Roll out to the needed size and thickness.
(*Alternatively, you can Flour the work surface along with the rolling pin. This method will require a great deal of Flour on both the rolling pin and on the work surface. It may also dry out the Dough resulting in a more crumbly finish*)

NOTES:

SAUCES

Basic White Sauce
"Bechamel"

1 Small	Yellow Onion
2 Cups	Milk
1	Bay Leaf
3 Tbs	White Rice Flour
3 Tbs	Butter
¼ tsp	Salt
¼ tsp	Black Pepper

Cut the Onion in half & peel only one half. Cut one (1) slice of onion from this half. Wrap up both remaining halves and refrigerate for some other use.

In a small sauce pan combine the Onion slice, Milk and Bay Leaf over medium heat. Slowly heat the milk until just bubbling, but not boiling. Remove from heat and let sit for about ten (10) minutes. Remove the Onion and Bay Leaf and cover the pan.

In a second sauce pan make a Roux by melting the butter over medium heat. Stir in the Rice Flour and whisk together. Stir constantly so the Roux doesn't brown. The mixture should begin to bubble, remove from heat and let it cool until the bubbling stops.

Pour the warm Milk into the Roux constantly whisking. Place pan back on the stove over medium heat. Keep whisking until the sauce is up to temperature then reduce heat to low. As the temperature lowers the sauce will thicken. Keep whisking.

Taste the sauce for flavor and texture. Add the Salt & Pepper to taste. Use immediately.

Cheese Sauce:	Add two (2) Cups of Shredded Cheese
Mornay Sauce:	Add ½ Cup Gruyere Cheese and ¼ Cup of Grated Parmesan whisking constantly.

Tips:

- White Pepper is more mild than Black Pepper and will not leave "specks" in the finished saucepan
- If you intend to hold the sauce more than an hour, lightly place small cubes of cold butter on the top of the sauce. As the sauce cools the Butter will prevent a skin from forming.
- Adding more Milk or Flour will thin or thicken the Roux as it cooks
- If making a Cheese sauce, don't add salt until after you've added all the cheese.

Bolognese Sauce

6 Slices	Thick Cut Bacon
1 Lb.	Sweet Italian Sausage
1 Lb.	Lean Ground Beef or Turkey
½ Cup	Onion, finely chopped
½ Cup	Carrot, finely chopped
½ Cup	Celery, finely chopped
¼ Cup	Butter
¼ Cup	Red Wine
3 Cloves	Fresh Garlic, minced
½ Tbs	Cinnamon
½ Tbs	Nutmeg
½ Tbs	Salt
½ Tbs	Ground Black Pepper
1 tsp	Oregano
1 tsp	Basil
½ Cup	Beef Stock
2 Tbs	Tomato Paste
12oz Can	Stewed Tomatoes
16oz Can	Tomato Sauce

Dice Bacon and saute in large, heavy stock pot over high heat. Once the Bacon has started to brown, add Sausage and Ground Meat. Cook for three(3) minutes stirring constantly. Add Butter, chopped Onion, Carrot and Celery and reduce heat to medium high stirring occasionally. Cook until the Onions are translucent and Carrots are soft.

Add the Red Wine and stir for one (1) minute loosening any bits of meat stuck to the bottom of the pot. Add the minced Garlic and cook for two(2) minutes. Sprinkle all the spices including the Salt & Pepper over ingredients and mix well. Let it cook for a few more minutes.

Stir in the Tomato Paste. Add the Beef Stock, Stewed Tomatoes and Tomato Sauce mixing well. Lower the heat to simmer and let cook for two(2) hours or more.

Serve over Gluten Free Spaghetti along with Gluten Free Garlic Bread.

Tips:

- If Sauce thickens too quickly, gradually add ¼ Cups of water to thin, but the finished product should be a thicker, heavier sauce than a plain Marinara.
- If Sauce is too thin add Tomato Paste one(1) Tablespoon at a time until it thickens.
- Just before serving, stir in ¼ Cup of Whipping Cream or Milk for a silky texture

Easy Hollandaise Sauce

1 Cup	**Butter**
4	**Eggs**
4 Tbs	**Hot Water**
3 tsp	**Lemon Juice**
¼ tsp	**Salt**
¼ tsp	**Ground Black Pepper**

Clarify the Butter (see Tips & Techniques section if needed)

Separate the Eggs (see Tips & Techniques section if needed)

In a Blender:
Pour Egg Yolks in blender and add the 3 Tbs of Water. Turn on blender and slowly pour Butter through the hole in the lid. Stop the blender to scrape down the sides and continue pulsing for another minute until combined and thickened.

Add Lemon Juice, Salt and Pepper. Pulse in short three (3) second intervals. Taste and adjust seasoning.

Ready to serve or hold in a sealed container for an hour or two. Serve over poached Eggs, poached Fish or steamed Veggies.

Tips:

- Serve Hollandaise Sauce just warmed, not hot. The other food served with it (ie. meat, fish, veggies) should be hot enough to heat the sauce further on contact.
- Strain the sauce through a mesh sieve to remove any bits the blender missed and ensure a smooth finish if needed.
- The traditional method would be to whisk the sauce over a double-boiler instead of using a blender. The traditional method requires more skill and focus.

This pasta sauce is super easy and tasty. You can whip this sauce up to use right away in a pinch for Chicken Parmesan or Meatballs. However, it's best after it simmers for a few hours and is even better when reheated the next day! - DPS

Simple Spaghetti Sauce

4	**Fresh Roma Tomatoes**
2 Cans	**Whole Tomatoes**
2 Cans	**Stewed Tomatoes**
1 Can	**Tomato Sauce**
1 Can	**Tomato Paste**
2 Cloves	**Fresh Garlic (Chopped)**
1 Medium	**Yellow Onion (Diced)**
1 Cup	**Chicken Stock**
¼ Cup	**Sugar**
2 Cup	**Water**
2 Tbs	**Oregano**
1 Tbs	**Basil**
1 Tbs	**Salt**
1 Tbs	**Pepper**
¼ Cup	**Olive Oil**
3 Tbs	**Butter**

Rinse Roma Tomatoes and quarter. Set aside.

In a large stock pot warm Olive Oil and melt Butter over medium/high heat. Sauté Onions for approximately 3 minutes. Add Garlic and continue to sauté 3 more minutes. Squeeze Roma Tomato quarters by hand over pot and place in the pot cooking 2 minutes.

Add Whole Tomatoes and Stewed Tomatoes cooking 3 minutes. Add Tomato Sauce, Oregano, Basil, Salt & Pepper. Add Chicken Stock and Sugar. Add Water and reduce temperature to low to simmer 4-6 hours.

Our kids love this recipe with Chicken, Pork Chops and stir fry dinners. The seasoning can be adjusted to make it more or less sweet depending on your taste. "Mirin" is a Japanese sweet seasoning made from Rice Alcohol. It can usually be found in any supermarket's Asian section. -DPS

Homemade Teriyaki Sauce

2 Cups	**Gluten-Free Soy Sauce**
¾ Cup	**Light Brown Sugar**
¾ Cup	**Sugar**
Half	**Small Onion**
2 tsp	**Fresh Ginger, minced**
1	**Fresh Garlic Clove, minced**
2 Tbs	**Mirin**
1 Cup	**Honey**

Peel and slice Onion and place in a sauce pan. Add the Soy Sauce and bring up to temperature over medium high heat. Add the Ginger and Garlic and stir.

When the sauce just begins to boil add both of the Sugars. Stir with a whisk to combine completely and reduce heat to a low simmer.

Add the Mirin and Honey stirring to incorporate. Increase the heat to high and bring to a boil. The mixture should foam quickly. Once it does remove the pan from the heat and let cool. With a slotted spoon remove the Onion slices and pour sauce into a seal-able container.

Keep refrigerated.

These are two of our favorite accompaniments to seafood dishes. Simple recipes that add a fresh and great flavor to seafood! - DPS

Shrimp Cocktail Sauce

1 Cup	Ketchup
1 tsp	Minced Horseradish
1 tsp	Lemon Juice, fresh
½ tsp	Sugar
½ tsp	Black Pepper

Combine all ingredients in a bowl and whisk together. Taste and adjust seasonings if needed.

Basic Tartar Sauce

1 Cup	Mayonnaise
2 Tbs	Dill Pickle, chopped
1 Tbs	Onion, grated
2 tsp	Lemon Juice, fresh
1 tsp	Tarragon
½ tsp	Salt

Chop the Dill Pickle and place in a small bow. Grate the Onion and add to the bowl. Combine all the remaining ingredients and stir well.

Cover and refrigerate for an hour before using.

My favorite part of barbecuing is making the Rub and the Sauce. This recipe comes from a number of other recipes we've tried over the years and adjusted to our taste. Leaving out the Liquid Smoke will give a more sweet flavor. - DPS

Basic Barbecue Sauce

2 Cups	Ketchup
¼ Cup	Apple Cider Vinegar
¼ Cup	Worcestershire Sauce
¼ Cup	Light Brown Sugar
2 Tbs	Molasses
2 Slices	Sweet Yellow Onion
2	Fresh Garlic Cloves
2 Tbs	Paprika
1 Tbs	Dry Mustard
1 tsp	Salt
1 tsp	Black Peppercorn
2 tsp	Liquid Smoke

Peel a small Yellow Onion and slice in half. Cut two(2) thick slices from one half and place in a saucepan. Save the remaining Onion for another use.

Add all ingredients to the saucepan and bring slowly to a boil. Reduce the heat and simmer on low for about an hour. Stir occasionally. The sauce will thicken and reduce while simmering.

Remove the Onion and Garlic Cloves and discard.
Store the sauce in glass jar. Keep refrigerated until needed.

Quick Pesto Sauce

2 Cups	Fresh Basil
2	Fresh Garlic Cloves
½ Cup	Virgin Olive Oil
1/3 Cup	Pine Nuts, toasted
1/3 Cup	Parmesan Cheese
	Salt & Pepper to season

If the Pine Nuts are not already toasted, preheat the oven to 375 degrees. Lay the Pine Nuts on a cookie sheet and bake in the oven ten (10) minutes or until the Pine Nuts are a light golden brown. Check every three (3) minutes and stir.

Wash and stem the Fresh Basil. Pat dry. In a food processor add the Basil. Peel the Garlic and add to the Basil. Place the cover on the food processor with the lid to the feed tube removed.

Begin slowly pouring the Olive Oil through the feed tube while pulsing the Basil and Garlic. Taste and add a pinch of Salt & Pepper.

Continue pulsing until the Pesto is smooth. When finished, pour into a medium size bowl.

Add the toasted Pine Nuts and the Parmesan Cheese. Mix well with a spoon.

Cover the bowl with a tight sealed lid and refrigerate until needed.

TIPS:

- The quickest way to toast Pine Nuts would be in a skillet. However, they can spot/burn easily and it requires your full attention while toasting.
- Walnuts are a great alternative to Pine Nuts

- Freshly grated Parmigiano-Reggiano is the best cheese to use for any Italian dish calling for Parmesan cheese. It is more expensive and very pungent so a little goes a long way.

NOTES:

BREADS

French Baguette

3 Cups	**All Purpose Gluten Free Flour**
2 Tbs	**Sugar**
2 Tbs	**Active Dry Yeast**
2 Tbs	**Xanthum Gum**
1 tsp	**Salt**
3	**Eggs**
1	**Egg White**
2 Tbs	**Butter, melted**
1 tsp	**Cider Vinegar**
1 ½ Cup	**Water, Very Warm**

Keep a small, extra amount of flour available to add during the mixing process.

In a mixing bowl add all the dry ingredients stirring together.

Crack two (2) eggs into a large bowl. Add the melted Butter and whisk together. Add the Cider Vinegar and the warm Water and whisk lightly.

With the mixer set on a low setting begin pouring the wet ingredients until combined. The dough should appear more like a sticky batter at this point. Begin adding some extra flour by the tablespoon until the dough begins to thicken around the paddle.

Add the Egg White and mix for one (1) minute. Set aside to let it rest. Prepare the pan(s). Either grease the pan with cooking spray or use parchment paper.

The dough will be very light and moist. Pour the dough into a plastic bag and clip one corner to make a "tip." Twist the closed end of the bag to force the dough through the makeshift tip onto the pan(s) in the shape of a loaf, twelve (12) inches or more.

Wet your hands and softly smooth out the loaves until they are even. Whisk the last Egg in a small bowl with a teaspoon of water to make an Egg Wash. Very lightly brush the loaves with the Egg Wash.

Set in a warm, humid place to rise (approximately 25-35 minutes).

Preheat oven to 400 degrees Fahrenheit

Place a cookie sheet or small ovenproof pan in the oven while preheating. Remove the loaves from the proofing area and bake for forty (40) minutes. Toss a handful of ice cubes onto the cookie sheet to create steam for the bread. This will give it a crisp crust.

Place finished bread on a cooling rack to cool.

A good Potato Roll or Hamburger Bun is perfect for any Barbecue items, especially Burgers or Pulled Pork Sliders! Enjoy! - DPS

Potato Hamburger Buns

2 Cups	**All Purpose Gluten Free Flour**
1 Cup	**Potatoes, precooked & mashed**
2 Tbs	**Sugar**
2 Tbs	**Active Dry Yeast**
2 Tbs	**Xanthum Gum**
1 tsp	**Salt**
4	**Eggs**
1	**Egg White**
4 Tbs	**Butter, melted**
1 tsp	**Cider Vinegar**
1 ½ Cup	**Water, Very Warm**

Keep a small, extra amount of flour available to add during the mixing process.

In a mixing bowl add all the dry ingredients, including the Potatoes stirring together.

Crack three (3) eggs into a large bowl. Add the melted Butter and whisk together. Add the Cider Vinegar and the warm Water and whisk lightly.

With the mixer set on a low setting begin pouring the wet ingredients until combined. The dough should appear more like a sticky batter at this point. Begin adding some extra flour by the tablespoon until the dough begins to thicken around the paddle.

Add the Egg White and mix for one (1) minute. Set aside to let it rest.

Spoon the dough onto a greased baking sheet. Wet your hands and form the dough into a bun shape.

Whisk the last Egg in a small bowl with a teaspoon of water to make an Egg Wash. Very lightly brush the buns with the Egg Wash. Set in a warm, humid place to rise (approximately 25-35 minutes).

Preheat oven to 400 degrees Fahrenheit

Remove the buns from the proofing area and bake for twenty (20) minutes or until golden brown. Place individually on a rack to cool.

To me, the key ingredient to a good NAAN is the Plain Yogurt. It brings a new dimension to the flavor with it's creaminess and by allowing the Butter to really stand out in the finished product. We love this bread toasted and dipped in Mint Hummus and for sandwiches or just as a yummy snack! - DPS

Flatbread or NAAN

2 Cups	**Water, very warm**
3 Tbs	**Instant Dry Yeast**
2 Tbs	**Sugar**
1 ½ tsp	**Salt**
½ Cup	**Extra Virgin Olive Oil**
4 Tbs	**Plain Yogurt**
¼ Cup	**Butter, melted**
1	**Egg**
4 Cups	**All-Purpose GFree Flour**
1 tsp	**Dry Gelatin**

In a small bowl whisk the Yeast in the Water. The Water should be warm, but not hot. Allow the Yeast to proof in the water. It should begin to foam. If not, discard and start over.

Once the Yeast foams whisk in the Olive Oil, Sugar and Salt.

In a mixing bowl combine the Yogurt, Butter and Egg and mix until well blended. Add the liquid Yeast mixture and continue mixing. Add the Flour and beat on medium speed for three (3) minutes. Add the Gelatin and beat another minute. Remove the bowl from the mixer, cover with a warm, damp cloth and let rise for thirty 30 minutes.

Cut two (2) even strips of Parchment Paper. Lay one (1) sheet on a flat surface and grease with cooking spray.

Scoop Bread batter and spread on greased parchment paper leaving room to roll into mini-loaves. Grease the second piece of parchment paper with cooking spray and lay greased side on top of batter drops. Roll each batter drop to approximately four (4) inches round. Leave space for mini-loaves to rise. Cover and let rise for thirty (30) minutes.

Preheat oven to 325 degrees.

Bake for twenty (20) minutes or until golden brown. Remove from oven and cool on a cooling rack.

Reheat in the oven, pan fried in hot oil or grilled before serving.

Is there anything better than warm Banana Bread with a pad of butter melting on it? Our kids love, love, love this recipe and request it often! - DPS

Quick & Easy Banana Bread

1 1/3 Cup	**All-Purpose Gluten Free Flour**
¾ Cup	**Butter, softened**
1 Cup	**Granular Sugar**
1	**Egg**
1 Cup	**Ripe Bananas, peeled & mashed**
2 Tbs	**Sour Cream**
½ Cup	**Chopped Walnuts**
½ tsp	**Baking Powder**
½ tsp	**Baking Soda**

Preheat oven to 350 degrees.

Grease a standard bread pan from the entire bottom, all the way to the top of each side.

In a mixing bowl cream the Butter on medium speed. Add the Sugar, then Egg and continue beating. The mix should start to lighten and become fluffy. If not, increase speed of the mixer.

Shut off mixer and scrape down the sides of the bowl. Add all the remaining ingredients. Mix on medium speed until all the ingredients are combined. The consistency should be thick and wet like a cake batter.

Pour into the greased bread pan and bake for one hour.

Gently remove from oven and allow to fully cool before cutting.

SALADS

Antipasto Salad

¼ Lbs	**Salami, thin sliced**
¼ Lbs	**Provolone Cheese, sliced**
2 Large	**Green Peppers**
1 Large	**Red Peppercorn**
½ Lb	**Fresh Mushrooms**
½ Lb	**Grape Tomatoes**
1 Small	**Onion**
¼ Cup	**Black Olives, pitted**
¼ Cup	**Olive Oil**
2 Tbs	**Red Wine Vinegar**
1 Tbs	**Basil**
1 Tbs	**Oregano**
1 Tbs	**Parsley**

Salt & Pepper to taste

Preheat oven to 375 degrees.

Cut each Pepper in half to remove the seeds and ribs. Lightly Salt and place in a small roasting pan. Roast in the oven for ten (10) minutes or just until they start to soften.

Remove from the oven and allow to cool. When the Peppers are cooled lay on a cutting board with the cut side down. Slice the Pepper in half. Then in half again. Repeat one more time so each Pepper half has been cut into eight (8) strips.

Clean the mushrooms and pat dry. cut in half if they are large. Remove the skin of the Onion and cut into quarters. Then cut each quarter in half.
In a medium size bowl add the Mushrooms, Onions and Tomatoes. Pour the Olive Oil and Red Wine Vinegar over the vegetables. Add the Basil, Oregano and Parsley. With a large spoon gently turn the vegetables until they are coated with the oil and seasoning.

On a large plate fan all the Pepper slices in a circle starting from the center of the plate. Spoon the marinated vegetables over the fanned Peppers starting from the center of the plate.

Roll each slice of Salami and each slice of Provolone. Place on the outer edge of the plate alternating meat and cheese between each Pepper slice. Dot the plate with the Black Olives.

Serve with a warm, sliced Baguette.

Basic Cole Slaw

1	**Head Cabbage**
4	**Large Carrots**
¼	**Small Onion**
½ Cup	**Mayo**
¼ Cup	**Butter Milk**
¼ Cup	**Fat-Free Milk**
1/3 Cup	**White Sugar**
2 ½ Tbs	**Lemon Juice**
1 ½ Tbs	**White Vinegar**
1 tsp	**Salt**

Shred or Chop Cabbage into strings approximately 2 inches or longer. Place in a mixing bowl.

Shred the Carrots and place in the bowl.

Chop Onion into fine bits and add to the bowl.

Add the remaining ingredients together in a smaller separate bowl. Whisk together until combined.

Pour over the vegetables and mix well.

Cover and refrigerate for 4-5 hours.

This is a variation of a recipe my wife used for years before we went Gluten Free. We bring this salad to Barbecues and it's always a big hit! This is one of those dishes that your guests won't believe is Gluten Free! - DPS

Summer Time Penne Salad

1 Pckg	**Gluten Free Penne**
¼ Cup	**Sun Dried Tomatos,chopped**

Dressing:

¼ Cup	**Red Wine Vinegar**
1/3 Cup	**Olive Oil**
2 Cloves	**Fresh Garlic (minced)**

4 tsp	**Spicy Brown Mustard**
2 T	**Lemon Juice**
½ tsp	**Thyme(fresh or dried)**
1 tsp	**Dill Weed**

Salt & Pepper to Taste

Bring 4 quarts of water to a boil and pour in pasta. While stirring occasionally, cook the pasta until *Al Dente* ("to the bite") which is typically One (1) minute less than directions on the package.

While Penne is cooking in a medium size bowl mix dressing ingredients with a whisk or fork. Set aside

Place a colander in the sink to drain the pasta. Briefly rinse with cool water and let sit for five (5) minutes. After five (5) minutes, rinse again to remove any starch and place into a large mixing bowl.

Pour dressing over pasta reserving an ounce or two for later. Add the Sun Dried Tomatoes. With two large spoons very gently mix and toss to combine. Cover, place in the refrigerator to cool.

Remove from the refrigerator 20 minutes before serving and add remaining salad dressing. Toss lightly and serve

Tips:

- This salad is best if left to stand and cool for a few hours before serving.
- For more flavor add bite sized: Black Olives, Cucumber, Cherry or Grape Tomatoes, Garbanzo Beans, etc.

This is our version of a recipe we found over twenty years ago. We always seem to pair it with seafood dishes, but it truly goes with just about anything. As they say "Bacon makes everything better!" - DPS

Warm Spinach Salad

1 LB	**Fresh Spinach**
4 Strips	**Hickory Smoked Bacon**
¼ Cup	**Red Onion – sliced**
1 Cup	**Fresh Mushrooms**
2	**Fresh Garlic Cloves**
1 tsp	**Dijon Mustard**
1 tsp	**Sugar**
4 oz	**Red Cooking Wine**
6 oz	**Olive Oil**

Wash and Stem the Spinach then pat dry. Chop into large, rough pieces and put in a bowl.

Dice the Bacon and cook in a saute pan until it just begins to crisp.

Dice the Mushrooms, slice the Red Onion and mince the Garlic while the Bacon is cooking.

Pour off half the Bacon grease and add the Onions, Garlic and Mushrooms to the pan cooking for two minutes. Pour the Bacon and veggies in a bowl and set aside.

Increase the heat, add Vinegar or Sherry to the pan scraping with a wooden spoon or spatula to loosen the tiny bits and deglaze it. After a minute or so, add the Olive Oil, Dijon Mustard and Sugar to the pan. Stir to blend.

Add the Bacon and veggies to the Spinach and pour the hot glaze over it all.

Toss lightly and serve immediately.

Tuna-Mac Salad

2 Cups	GFree Macaroni Shells
1	Tuna Fish
6	Hard-Boiled Eggs
1 Cup	Celery
1 Cup	Mayo
1	Green Onion
½ tsp	Dry Mustard
¼ tsp	Salt
¼ tsp	Black Pepper
½ tsp	Parsley
Garnish	Paprika

Cook the Macaroni one (1) minute less than the directions on the package for Al Dente. Rinse and cool before mixing in the salad.

Pour the Macaroni in a large mixing bowl. Add Mayo, and dry mustard. Mix well. Chop Celery and Green Onion, add to the bowl.

Open the can of Tuna Fish and drain well, add to the bowl.

Set aside 5 slices of the Egg and chop remainder, add to the bowl. Mix well.

Add Salt & Pepper to taste.

Place salad into a serving bowl. Arrange the saved Egg slices in a circle on top of the salad

Dust top of the salad with Paprika and sprinkle with fresh Parsley

Cover & place in the refrigerator for 2-3 hours to cool.

Store bought Gluten Free Tortellini is very delicate. It can often come apart (i.e. "unroll") or end up very mushy when cooking so be very gentle. This is a dish you should practice a few times before you offer it to guests. - DPS

Tortellini Salad

1 Pckg	Gluten Free Tortellini

Dressing:

¼ Cup	Red Wine Vinegar
1/3 Cup	Olive Oil
2 Cloves	Fresh Garlic, minced

4 tsp	Spicy Brown Mustard
2T	Lemon Juice
½ tsp	Thyme(fresh or dried)
1 tsp	Dill Weed (fresh or dried)

1/8 tsp	Ground Black Pepper
½ tsp	Salt

Bring 4 quarts of water to a boil and gently pour in Tortellini. While stirring occasionally, cook the pasta until *Al Dente* ("to the bite") which is typically one (1) minute less than directions on the package.

While Tortellini is cooking in a medium size bowl mix dressing ingredients with a whisk or fork. Set aside

Place a colander in the sink and slowly drain the pasta. Briefly rinse with cool water and let sit for five (5) minutes. After five (5) minutes, rinse briefly again and place into a large mixing bowl.

Pour dressing over pasta reserving an ounce or two for later. With two large spoons very carefully mix and toss to combine. Cover, place in the refrigerator to cool.

Remove from the refrigerator 20 minutes before serving and add remaining salad dressing. Toss lightly and serve

TIPS:

- This salad is best if left to stand and cool for a few hours before serving.
- For more flavor add bite sized vegetables such as: Black Olives, Cucumber, Cherry or Grape Tomatoes, Sun Dried Tomatoes, Garbanzo Beans, etc.

Zesty Avocado Salad

2	**Fresh Avocado (Ripe)**
1	**Fresh Green Leaf Lettuce**
1	**Radicchio Lettuce**
15	**Leaves of Fresh Spinach**
½	**Large Red Onion**
15-20	**Cherry or Grape Tomatoes**
1	**Bunch Fresh Cilantro**
½ Cup	**Fresh Lime Juice**
¼ Cup	**Olive Oil**
1 Tbs	**Lime Zest**
½ tsp	**Sea Salt**
½ tsp	**Black Pepper**

Slice the Avocados in half and remove the pits. Remove the Avocado from the skin, keeping as much intact as possible. Slice each half along the short side and set aside.

Chop the Green Leaf, Radicchio and Spinach and place in a serving bowl. Peel the Red Onion and slice thinly along the short side. Place in the bowl.

Rinse Tomatoes and pat dry. If the Tomatoes seem extra large, slice in half. Place all Tomatoes in the bowl.

In a food processor or blender add the following:

Rinse the fresh Cilantro and remove stems after you pat dry. Set aside a small handful. Put remaining Cilantro in the processor.

Add the remaining ingredients to the processor and pulse until it's pureed.

Drizzle a small amount over the salad ingredients and gently toss. Slowly add more dressing and toss until well combined.

Arrange slices of Avocado in a circle on top of the salad.

Sprinkle remaining Cilantro on Avocado.

APPETIZERS

Hot Artichoke Dip

½ Cup	Mayonnaise
½ Cup	Sour Cream
1 Can (14oz)	Artichoke Hearts
1/3 Cup	Parmesan Cheese Shredded
2	Garlic Cloves
1 Dash	Hot Sauce

Preheat oven to 350 degrees.

Drain Artichoke hearts and chop.

Chop or mince the Garlic cloves into small granules.

In a medium size bowl add Mayonnaise and Sour Cream stirring to mix. Add the Artichoke Hearts, Garlic and Parmesan.

Pour the dip in a baking dish leaving a small amount of Parmesan Cheese for topping.

Bake for 30 minutes.

Take the dish out of the oven and sprinkle the remaining Parmesan Cheese over the top and return to the oven for 10 more minutes or until cheese topping is melted.

Serve warm with Gluten Free Naan cut into triangles or corn tortilla chips.

Bruschetta

3	**Roma Tomatoes**
2	**Fresh Garlic Cloves**
12	**Fresh Basil Leaves**
¼ Cup	**Virgin Olive Oil**
Salt & Pepper to taste	

1 Loaf	**Gluten Free Baguette**

Preheat oven to 375 degrees.

Peel and mince the Garlic Cloves and place in a bowl with the Olive Oil.

Slice the Baguette into ¼ inch thick slices. Place the slices on a baking sheet and brush with the Garlic infused Olive Oil. Bake for three (3) minutes. Remove from the oven and flip each slice over and brush with Olive Oil. Return to the oven and cook until toasted lightly brown.
Remove from the oven and set aside.

Dice and seed the Roma Tomatoes. Place in to a medium size bowl. Pour the remaining Garlic infused Olive Oil over the Tomatoes.

Stack six (6) Basil leaves on top of each other. Roll tightly into the shape of a cigar. Holding the rolled leaves begin thinly slicing the leaf. Repeat with the remaining leaves and add to the bowl with the Tomatoes and Garlic.

Toss gently and season with Salt & Pepper.

Arrange the toasted bread on a plate and top with the Tomato mixture.

Serve immediately.

TIPS:

- Leave the bread on the baking sheet when adding the Tomatoes. Grate fresh Parmesan and return to the oven to melt the cheese for a heartier version of this crowd pleaser.

Classic Spinach Dip

1 Cup	**Mayo**
16oz	**Sour Cream**
10oz	**Frozen Chopped Spinach**
2	**Scallions**
1 Tbs	**Celery Salt**
1 Tbs	**Onion Powder**
½ tsp	**Salt**
¼ tsp	**Paprika**

Optional:

5oz	**Sliced Water Chestnuts**
2oz	**Shredded Carrot**

Drain Spinach and squeeze out excess water. Set aside.

Chop Scallions and Water Chestnuts(if using). Blend all the ingredients in a bowl. The Paprika can be overpowering so add a little at a time and taste.

Adjust the seasonings to your family's tastes.

For best results refrigerate for 3+ hours.

Serve with vegetable sticks and/or Gluten Free Baguette.

Cocktail Sausages or Meatballs

| 1 LB | "Smokies" Sausage or basic GF Meatballs (see below) |

Sauce

1/3 Cup	Chili sauce
1/3 Cup	Black or Red Currant Jam
1 TB	Lemon Juice
1 tsp	Dijon Mustard

Gluten Free Meatballs - basic

1 LB	Ground Beef
¼ Cup	Finely Chopped Onion
1	Egg
1 TB	Salt
1 TB	Black Pepper
¼ Cup	GF Bread Crumbs
1 tsp	Oregano
1 tsp	Basil
1 Tbs	Butter

For the Sauce: Combine Chili Sauce and Currant Jam in a stove top pan and bring up to medium heat. Add the Dijon Mustard and Lemon Juice. Simmer on low for 15 minutes.

For the Meatballs: Combine all ingredients in a bowl. Using a one (1oz) ounce ice cream scoop or tablespoon, scoop mixture onto a plate. Roll each scoop into a tight ball. Set aside.

Melt butter in a large frying pan and brown meatballs. Place browned Meatballs or Sausages in the sauce and simmer 20 minutes more.

Transfer to a crock-pot/slow-cooker and keep on low until you serve.

Crab Salad Cups

½ Lb	**Pre-Cooked Crab Meat**
1	**Fresh Mango**
6	**Fresh Scallions**
2 TBS	**Fresh Cilantro**
1	**Fresh Lime**
4 TBS	**Olive Oil**
15-18	**GFree Won-ton Wrappers**

Preheat oven to 375 degrees

Grease a muffin tin with cooking spray or shortening.

Brush both sides of each Won-ton Wrapper with the Olive Oil and gently press into muffin tin to form the cups. Bake until lightly browned, but crispy (approximately 8-10min). Let cool and remove carefully from the muffin tin.

Peel the Mango and begin slicing around the pit. Dice the Mango slices to small bite size portions. Place into a medium size mixing bowl.

Chop Scallions into small bite size portions and add to the bowl.

Chop fresh Cilantro and add to the bowl.

Add the Crab Meat to the bowl tossing gently.

In a small bowl grate the lime skin for the zest. Cut the lime in half, place a fork in the center of one

half and squeeze the juice out of the lime. Repeat with other lime half.
Add remaining Olive Oil to the lime and whisk together. Salt & Pepper to taste.
Pour over the Crab Meat and gently toss.

Spoon Crab Salad into each Won-ton and serve immediately or chill for later use.

TIPS:

- Add 1 tsp of finely diced Fresh Jalapeño or Dried Red Pepper flakes for some zip!
- If making ahead of time take the chilled salad cups out to allow to come to room temperature before serving.

Fresh Salsa

3	**Fresh Roma Tomatoes**
1	**Fresh Jalapeno Chile**
½	**Medium White Onion**
1	**Garlic Clove**
¼ Cup	**Fresh Cilantro**
1	**Lime**
½ tsp	**Salt**

Quarter the Roma Tomatoes and remove seeds. Place in a Food Processor.

Quarter the Jalapeno Chile. To remove the seeds and ribs, lay a Jalapeno quarter flat, skin side down. With the tip of a small, easy to handle sharp knife, cut the ribs & seeds in one stroke. Set aside seeds and ribs for additional seasoning later. Dice the Jalapeno and place in the Food Processor.

Chop the Onion. Place in the Food Processor.

Unwrap the Garlic Clove and chop roughly. Place in the Food Processor.

Using a Zester, scrape about a quarter of the Lime skin into the Food processor. Cut lime in half and squeeze the juice into the Food Processor.

Remove the Cilantro leaves from the stem and place leaves in the Food Processor.

Add half the Salt.

Pulse until well blended. Taste the Salsa. Adjust seasoning by adding Jalapeno ribs or additional Salt.

Transfer to a serving dish, cover with plastic and refrigerate for one (1) hour.

Serve cold, garnished with Fresh Cilantro.

TIPS:

- This Salsa is totally fresh so it's best to eat the same day.
- Add diced Peaches, Mango or Pineapple for a "Sweet & Spicy" finish.
- Stick a fork into the Lime as you squeeze the Lime to get additional juice. Don't let any Lime seeds get in the Food Processor.

Guacamole Dip

2	Avocado
2 Cups	Homemade Tomato Salsa
2 Tbs	Fresh Cilantro
1	Garlic Clove
1 Tbs	Lime Juice
¼ tsp	Sea Salt
¼ tsp	Ground Black Pepper
½ tsp	Ground Cumin

Cut Avocado in half and remove pit. Scoop Avocado out of skin into the bowl and mash with a fork into a paste.

Mince Garlic Clove and add to the bowl. Pour Lime juice over the Avocado. Add the Ground Cumin and mix well. Add the Tomato Salsa and fresh Cilantro and mix. Salt and Pepper to taste.

Cover and refrigerate for about an hour.

TIPS:

- If possible, take the Guacamole Dip out of the refrigerator with enough time to bring to room temperature.

Classic Hummus

2 Cups	**Chick Peas**
¼ Cup	**Tahini**
1.5 tsp	**Sea Salt**
3	**Garlic Cloves (minced)**
½ Cup	**Vegetable Oil**
	(keep ¼ Cup in reserve)
¼ Cup	**Lemon Juice**

Drain Chickpeas & rinse under cold water until clear then pat dry with paper towels.

Place all the ingredients in a food processor or blender and puree for 30 seconds. Stop machine and scrape down sides with a spatula. Add more Oil if the mixture seems dry and too thick.

Puree for an additional 20-30 seconds.

Add more salt or lemon juice to taste.

Yields 2 ½ Cups.

TIPS:

- For more variety add one or more of the following:
    Roasted Garlic
    Roasted Red Pepper
    Diced Jalapeno Pepper

Mint Hummus

1 Can	**Chick Peas**
1.5 tsp	**Sea Salt**
3	**Garlic Cloves minced**
½ Cup	**Vegetable Oil**
	(keep ¼ Cup in reserve)
¼ Cup	**Fresh Lemon Juice**
2 Tbs	**Fresh Mint Leaves**

Drain Chickpeas & rinse under cold water until clear then pat dry with paper towels.

Place all the ingredients in a food processor or blender and puree for 30 seconds. Stop machine and scrape down sides with a spatula. Add more Oil if the mixture seems dry and too thick.

Puree for an additional 20-30 seconds.

Add more Salt or Lemon Juice to taste.

Yields 2 cups.

TIPS:

- This particular recipe does not include Tahini. Please see Classic Hummus recipe for a more traditional Hummus.
- Do not use Lemon Juice from concentrate because the flavor cannot overcome the Peas, Garlic and Mint.

Stuffed Grape Leaves

1 Jar	**Grape Leaves**
1 ½ lb	**Ground Lamb or Beef**
1 Cup	**Rice (cooked)**
1 28oz Can	**Chopped Tomatoes**
1 28oz Can	**Chicken Stock**
	(see "Extra Stuff" section)
1 Large	**White Onion**
¼ tsp	**Cinnamon**
¼ tsp	**Sea Salt**
¼ tsp	**Black Pepper**

Follow directions on package to cook 1 cup of Rice.
Mix Meat with Rice, Salt, Pepper, the Cinnamon
and pulp of the Tomatoes(reserve juice for later).

Gently remove all the Grape Leaves from the jar
and rinse well to remove the brine. Line the bottom
of a 5 quart pot with Grape Leaves. Torn or smaller
leaves are perfect for the lining.

Lay a single Grape Leaf flat. Place a tablespoon of
the Meat mixture at the bottom of the Leaf leaving
an inch for rolling. Lift bottom of the Leaf and roll
once towards the top of the Leaf. Fold in each side.
Continue rolling until the entire Leaf is rolled
looking like a small cigar. Continue with each
Grape Leaf until all the Leaves or the Meat are
gone.

Lay the stuffed Leaves in the pot on top of the lining. Pour Chicken Stock and reserved Tomato Juice over the Leaves. Peel and slice the Onion in ¼ inch rings. Lay the Onions over the Leaves and cover. Bring to a boil and immediately reduce to low heat. Let simmer one hour.

TIPS:

- Sprinkle ½ teaspoon of fresh chopped Mint over the liquid prior to boiling.

Sausage Stuffed Mushrooms

24	**Whole, Fresh Mushrooms**
1 Lb	**Sweet Italian Sausage**
1 Cup	**GFree Bread Crumbs**
1 Stick	**Butter**
1 Small	**Yellow Onion**
2 Cloves	**Fresh Garlic (minced)**
1/3 Cup	**Shredded Parmesan**

Preheat oven to 375 Degrees

Rinse Mushrooms and pat dry with towel (cloth or paper). Pull stems from each Mushroom and set aside.

Line baking dish with Mushroom Caps. Dice Mushroom Stems and set aside in a bowl. Dice Onion and add to the bowl with Mushroom stems. Add fresh minced Garlic.

Heat on high a non-stick frying pan and place Italian Sausage in pan with the Butter. Reduce heat to medium-high and saute Sausage until cooked through. Add the bowl with Stems, Garlic and Onions to the Sausage and saute for two minutes.

Add Gluten Free Bread Crumbs to the pan and mix all ingredients thoroughly. If the ingredients are too dry, add a small amount of melted Butter or a small Egg to moisten.

Stuff each Mushroom Cap with mixture.

Bake in the oven, uncovered for approximately 15-20 minutes or until Mushroom Caps are softened and cooked through.

Add Parmesan Cheese to the Mushroom Caps for the last five (5) minutes of cooking.

SIDES

Country Cauliflower

1 Large	Fresh Cauliflower
1 Cup	Sour Cream
4oz	Parmesan Cheese Shredded
2 tsp	Sesame Seeds

Salt & Pepper to taste

Preheat oven to 350 degrees

Chop Cauliflower into bite-size pieces. Bring 4 quarts of water to a boil. Place Cauliflower in the boiling water and cook until tender, approximately 6-7 minutes. Drain and rinse with cold water.

Place half of the cooked Cauliflower in a large baking or casserole dish. Spread half of the Sour Cream and half Parmesan Cheese on the top. Sprinkle with 1 tsp of Sesame Seeds.

For the second layer, place remaining half of the cooked Cauliflower on top. Spread the remaining Sour Cream and Parmesan over the Cauliflower. Sprinkle with the rest of the Sesame Seeds.

Bake uncovered for 5 minutes or until the cheese has melted and the casserole is heated through.

TIPS:
- Add three strips of chopped, crisp Bacon throughout both layers.

Creamy Mashed Potatoes

10	**Idaho Potatoes**
16oz	**Sour Cream**
8oz	**Softened Cream Cheese**
4 TB	**Butter**
3	**Garlic Cloves**
1 tsp	**Salt**
½ tsp	**Celery Salt**
1 tsp	**Ground Black Pepper**
	Paprika for garnish
	Chives for garnish

Peel and quarter the Potatoes. Place Potatoes in a pot (approximately 4 quarts) and cover with cold water. Add a teaspoon of Salt. Bring the water to a boil then reduce the heat to a low simmer. Cover and continue simmering on low for 20 minutes.

When a fork can easily cut through the Potatoes, they are done. Drain the water and briefly rinse with cool water. Drain again until the water is out of the pot. Mash briefly by hand with a potato masher.

Slice Butter into tablespoon size chunks and stir into the Potatoes. Add Sour Cream. Blend with a hand-held electric mixer on medium speed.

Mince the Garlic Cloves and add to the Potatoes. Combine all remaining ingredients in the pot.

Blend with hand-held mixer on medium speed until completely smooth. Increase the mixer speed to high to "whip" the Potatoes. Gently pour into a baking or casserole dish.

Sprinkle with Paprika until the entire casserole is dusted a light red color.

Sprinkle the center with a small amount of chives.

Warm in the oven until ready to serve.

Green Bean Casserole

1 ½ lbs	Green Beans
2 Tbs	GFree Flour
1 Cup	Fat-Free Milk
½ Cup	Shredded Swiss Cheese
½ Cup	Sour Cream
¼ Cup	Onion
1	Egg White
1 ½ Cup	GFree Croutons
4 Tbs	Butter or Margarine
1 tsp	Sugar
3 Tbs	Olive Oil
½ tsp	Oregano
½ tsp	Basil
½ tsp	Dried Garlic
2 Tbs	Grated Parmesan Cheese

Preheat oven to 350 degrees

See recipe for Gluten Free Croutons

Wash Green Beans and pat dry. Snap off ends and place in a casserole dish.

Place Croutons in a plastic bag and pound with a kitchen hammer to crush or grind in a food processor.

Melt 2 Tablespoons of Butter in a medium saucepan. Add Onions and sauté until tender.

Add Flour and stir until thickened. Add the milk while stirring constantly. Blend in Swiss Cheese, Sour Cream, Sugar and Salt. Cook 5 minutes stirring constantly.

Remove from heat and pour over Green Beans.

Combine the Gluten Free Croutons with 2 Tablespoons of melted butter and the egg white. Sprinkle over Green Beans.

Cook for 25 minutes at 350 degrees.

Cheezy Potatoes & Ham

6	**Medium Idaho Potatoes**
½ Lbs	**Honey Ham, sliced thick**
2 Tbs	**Butter**
4 Tbs	**Gluten Free Flour**
2 ½ Cups	**Cheddar Cheese, shredded**
¼ Cups	**Gorgonzola Cheese**
1 Cup	**Milk or Cream**

Preheat oven to 375 degrees

Set aside ½ Cup of the shredded Cheddar Cheese for the topping.

Slice the Ham in 2"x2" pieces. Set side. Slice the Potatoes either by hand or using a mandolin for thin, even pieces.

Layer the bottom of a baking dish with 1/3 the Potatoes. Lightly season the Potatoes with Salt & Pepper. Sprinkle half of the sliced Ham over the Potatoes. Add another 1/3 of Potatoes and then the remaining Ham. Top with the remaining Potatoes.

Next, make a Roux. In a saucepan melt the Butter. Add the Flour and whisk for one (1) minute to cook the Flour. Add half the Milk or Cream while stirring.

Begin adding the Cheddar Cheese by the handful. Stir until the Cheese is melted and fully blended. Continue add the Cheese until it is all in the saucepan. If the Sauce begins to thicken too much add some more Milk or Cream, but only enough to keep the sauce creamy.

Add the Gorgonzola and stir to incorporate. Slowly add remaining Milk or Cream. Stirring constantly.

Pour Cheese Sauce over the Potatoes and Ham.

Sprinkle the top of the dish with the ½ Cup of Shredded Cheddar Cheese.

Cover with foil and bake for 40-45 minutes or until the Potatoes are fork tender.

Remove the foil and broil under high heat for a few minutes to brown the Cheese topping.

TIPS:

- Substitute another strong flavored Cheese for the Gorgonzola
- Substitute Prosciutto for the Ham

Sometimes the simplest recipes are the most flavorful. This side dish is excellent in late summer when the Carrots and Mint Leaves are at their freshest. It's quick, it's easy and it is delicious! - DPS

Glazed Carrots

2 Cups	**Fresh Carrots**
2 Tbs	**Butter**
1 tsp	**Honey**
3 Tbs	**Fresh Mint Leaves**
¼ tsp	**Salt**

Peel Carrots and cut into 1-2 inch lengths. Set aside.

Wash and stem the Mint Leaves. Pat dry and place on a cutting board. Finely dice the Mint as small as possible.

In a saucepan melt the Butter over medium-high heat. Add the Honey and stir to incorporate. Add the Carrots and turn to coat.

Add the diced Mint leaves and turn to coat. Lower the heat and simmer for ten (10) minutes or until Carrots are softened to fork tender.

Sprinkle the Salt very lightly and remove from the heat.

Serve warm.

This side dish has become a holiday staple for our family. It pairs perfectly with Roasted Pork or Beef. It's also the only way we can get our kids to eat Brussels Sprouts. We just have to keep reminding them there is lotsa Bacon in that pan!! - DPS

Roasted Brussels Sprouts & Bacon

2 Lbs	Fresh Brussels Sprouts
6 Slices	Thick Cut Bacon
6	Medium Carrots
1 Cup	Parsnip, chopped
1	Medium Onion
¼ Cup	Olive Oil
2	Garlic Cloves
1 tsp	Oregano
1 tsp	Basil

Salt & Pepper to taste

Preheat oven to 375 degrees.

Stem and peel the Brussels Sprouts and place in a large bowl. Peel Carrots and cut into lengths of 1-2 inches. Add to the bowl with the Brussels Sprouts. Peel Parsnip and cut into cubes approximately the same size as the Brussels Sprouts and add to the bowl.

Pour Olive Oil over the vegetables in the bowl and begin turning with a large spoon to coat everything.

Sprinkle the Oregano, Basil along with the Salt & Pepper. Turn with a spoon again to coat.

Pour the coated vegetables into a large roasting pan.

Dice Bacon into small pieces and sprinkle over vegetables.

Chop Garlic and sprinkle over the vegetables.

Bake uncovered for forty (40) minutes or until all the vegetables are fork tender. The Brussels Sprouts may require more time depending on their size.

Serve warm.

Sweet Potato Casserole

8	Large Sweet Potatoes
½ Cup	Sugar
½ Cup	Milk
1/3 Cup	Melted Butter
1 tsp	Vanilla Extract
1 TB	Salt
2	Eggs

Topping

2 Tbs	Vermont Maple Syrup
1 Cup	Brown Sugar
1 Cup	Chopped Pecans
1 Cup	Shredded Coconut
1/3 Cup	GFree All Purpose Flour
1/3 Cup	Melted butter

Peel and quarter the potatoes. Place Potatoes in a pot (approximately 4 quarts) and cover with cold water. Add a teaspoon of Salt. Bring the water to a boil then reduce the heat to a low simmer. Cover and continue simmering on low for 20 minutes. When a fork can easily cut through the Potatoes, they are done. Drain the water and briefly rinse with cool water. Drain again until the water is out of the pot.

Preheat the oven to 350 degrees.

In the pot add the Maple Syrup, Sugar, Milk, Butter, Vanilla Extract, Salt and Pepper. Mash by hand with a potato masher and stir with a large spoon or use a hand-held mixer set to medium. Transfer to a baking dish or casserole pan.

In a smaller bowl stir the dry ingredients for the topping together. Add the melted Butter and mix well. Sprinkle over the top of the Potatoes.

Bake uncovered at 350 degrees for 25 minutes.

Serve warm.

Another easy summertime favorite. Sometimes we replace the Rice with Quinoa. These Stuffed Peppers are so big they could be a meal on their own! - DPS

Stuffed Peppers

4	**Large Green Peppers**
1 Lbs	**Ground Beef**
1	**Small Onion**
1 Cup	**Cooked Rice**
2	**Roma Tomatoes, very ripe**
2 Tbs	**Butter**
1 tsp	**Salt**
1 tsp	**Black Pepper**
¼ Cup	**Shredded Parmesan Cheese**

Paprika to season

Preheat oven to 350 degrees.

Cook the Rice according to the directions on the packet.

Cut off the tops of the Green Peppers to remove seeds and ribs. Cut a small amount of the bottoms, just enough so the Peppers will sit flat. Roast Green Peppers for fifteen (15) minutes. Remove from the oven, but leave on the cooking sheet to be stuffed and recooked.

Meanwhile, melt the better in a skillet. Add the Onion and saute until yellow. Add the Ground Beef.

Dice the Tomatoes and add to the skillet along with the juice. Season with Salt & Pepper.

Add the cooked Rice to the skillet and mix well.

Fill the Green Peppers with the mixture. Using a large spoon shape the mound of filling until smooth. Dust with Paprika.

Sprinkle the shredded Parmesan Cheese over each stuffed Pepper still on the baking sheet.

Return to the oven and bake another ten (10) minutes or until the Green Pepper is fork tender.

Increase the oven to a High Broil to brown the cheese (usually 30-40 seconds).

Stuffing or "Dressing"

2 Cups	**Gluten Free Bread Cubes**
4 Tbs	**Butter**
¼ Cup	**Fresh Parsley, chopped**
¼ Cup	**Celery, chopped**
¼ Cup	**Onion, chopped**
1 tsp	**Paprika**
½ tsp	**Nutmeg**
½ tsp	**Salt**
¼ Cup	**Chicken Stock**
	(see "Extra Stuff" section)

Melt the Butter in a saucepan. Add the Celery and Onion and saute until the Onion is Golden.

Add the cubed Bread and stir. Next, add the Fresh Parsley, the Paprika, Nutmeg and Salt. Continue stirring until the cubes and seasonings are well incorporated.

Slowly add the Chicken Stock to deglaze the pan and to moisten the Bread.

Transfer to a serving dish and garnish with sprigs of Parsley to serve.

Tips:
- If stuffing a Chicken or Turkey, omit the Chicken Stock.
- Adding Apples, Walnuts or Pecans to sweeten the dish.
- Gluten Free Croutons can be used instead, but you'll need to adjust the seasonings depending on the flavor of Crouton you use.

MAIN COURSES

Bourbon Chicken

2 Lbs	Boneless Chicken Breast

Marinade

½ Cup	Brown Sugar
½ Cup	Gluten Free Soy Sauce
½ Cup	Bourbon
2	Garlic Cloves (minced)
1 Tbs	Fresh Onion (minced)
1 tsp	Ground Ginger

2 Tbs	Virgin Olive Oil
2 Tbs	Butter
1	Small Onion
3 Tbs	White Cooking Wine

2 Cups	Cooked White Rice

Dice Chicken into 1-2 inch bites.

To make the Marinade, combine remaining ingredients, except White Wine and Onion, in a bowl. Stir to combine.

In a large plastic, resealable bag add Chicken and marinade. Refrigerate for 1-2 hours.

Cook Rice according to package directions and set aside.

Chop the Onion and set aside. Heat a large skillet to melt Butter and Olive Oil over high heat. Reduce the heat and add the Onion cooking for two (2) minutes.

Add marinated Chicken along with the marinade from the bag to the skillet. Cook for 2-3 minutes.

Add White Wine and cook another five (5) minutes or until the chicken is cooked through.

Serve over White Rice.

Lebanese Chicken & Rice Casserole

¼ Cup	**Olive Oil**
6 Lg	**Chicken Breasts**
3 Tbs	**Butter**
2 Medium	**Yellow Onions**
2 Cups	**Cooked White Rice**
24oz	**Chicken Stock**
1 tsp	**Cinnamon**
½ tsp	**Nutmeg**
¼ tsp	**Cumin**
1 tsp	**Salt**
1 tsp	**Ground Black Pepper**

Preheat oven to 325 degrees.

Slice the onions into large rings and set aside.

In a large sauce pan bring the Olive Oil to temperature on medium-high. Place Chicken Breasts in pan turning so they don't brown. Using tongs pull each piece of Chicken and quarter with a sharp knife. Return to pan and continue to stir while quartering the remaining breasts.

Add Butter, then the Onions to the pan and saute for two(2) minutes. Add the Chicken Stock to the sauce pan. Lower the heat to medium and continue cooking until Chicken is cooked through.

In a separate sauce pan cook the Rice according to the directions on the packet. You'll need two (2) Cups of cooked Rice for this recipe.

Remove each piece of Chicken and dice into bite sized pieces. Place in a Casserole dish. Add Rice to casserole dish and mix with the Chicken. Add all the seasonings to the dish and mix well. Taste and adjust spices to your satisfaction.

Lay the onion slices over the top of the dish. Bake, covered for 15 minutes.

TIPS:

- Add Butter and Ground Parmesan Cheese to the top for a crusty topping.
- Adding ground Cumin or Allspice will give the dish a more "earthy" flavor.
- Serve without placing in the oven for a more rustic meal.
- Sprinkle with roasted Pine Nuts for more flavor.

New England Chicken Cacciatore

1	**Whole Chicken (3-4LBS)**
¼ Cup	**Vegetable Oil**
1 Medium	**Yellow Onion, Diced**
2 Cloves	**Fresh Garlic**
16oz Can	**Whole Tomatoes**
½ Cup	**GF All PurposeFlour**
1 Cup	**Dry White Wine**
16oz Can	**Tomato Sauce**
16oz	**Chicken Stock**
	(see "Extra Stuff" section)
1 Tbs	**Oregano**
1 Tbs	**Basil**
½ tsp	**Celery Seed**
1 tsp	**Salt**
1 Tbs	**Ground Black Pepper**
2	**Bay Leaves**

Pour Vegetable Oil in a deep, heavy pan and heat on medium-high. While Oil is heating up, cut Chicken into pieces at each joint, leaving the bone in. Cut the breast into two (2) or three (3) even pieces.

Mix the Flour with the Salt & Pepper. Lightly dust the Chicken with the flour mixture.

Using tongs, add the Chicken into the Oil skin side down. Add the Onions. Once the pan is full of Chicken, the temperature will drop so increase the heat to get it back to temperature (approx 375F). Turn each piece after four (4) minutes and continue frying for five(5) minutes more.

Move Chicken to the side of the pan and pour in the Wine to deglaze. Let the alcohol burn off for about a minute.

Lower the heat and add the Fresh Garlic. Sauté until they just start to turn translucent. Pour the Tomatoes, Tomato Sauce and Stock over chicken. Add spices and stir. Cover & Simmer one (1) hour on low heat.

Remove cover and cook additional 15 minutes. Remove Bay Leaves, skim any fat that has risen to surface and serve over Gluten Free Pasta, Rice or in a bowl by itself.

TIPS:

- To make this dish "Italian Style" add Sliced Mushrooms and Kalamata Olives
- When adding the Wine don't pour over the meat. Pour directly on to the pan

Chicken Cordon Bleu

4	**Chicken Breast**
8	**Slices of Virginia Ham**
8	**Slices of Swiss Cheese**
4	**Slices of Provolone Cheese**
2 Cups	**GFree Bread Crumbs**
1 Tbs	**Salt**
1 Tbs	**Ground Black Pepper**
1 tsp	**Dried Oregano**
¼ Cup	**Vegetable Oil**
Toothpicks	

Preheat oven to 400 degrees.

Pour Gluten Free Bread Crumbs in a wide bowl.
Add Salt, Pepper and Oregano

On a cutting board slice each Chicken Breast
horizontally in half. Cover each Chicken Breast half
with plastic wrap and flatten with meat tenderizer
hammer. Place one slice of Ham on each Chicken
Breast. Layer with one slice of Swiss Cheese and
one half slice of Provolone.

From the end of the Chicken Breast begin rolling
until closed like a cigar. Place in the bowl of Gluten
Free Bread Crumbs and turn until completely
covered. Secure with toothpick or tie with kitchen
string if necessary.

In a large skillet bring Oil to medium-high heat. Using tongs add each rolled Chicken Breast to the skillet. Turn every 2-3 minutes. Place on a cookie sheet.

Bake at 400F for forty (40) minutes or until internal temperature is 165 degrees.

Check at twenty (20) minutes to ensure the cheese isn't pouring out of the ends.

Serve with steamed Veggies or Garlic Mashed Potatoes

TIPS:

- For a more crispy finish, fry each Chicken Breast again after they've baked in the oven
- Add an Egg Wash or Milk prior to the Bread Crumbs for a thicker breading.

Chicken Marsala

4	**Large Chicken Breast**
2 Cups	**White Rice Flour**
1 tsp	**Oregano**
1 tsp	**Basil**
1 tsp	**Black Peppercorn**
1 Cups	**Milk**
¼ Cup	**Olive Oil**
6 Tbs	**Butter**
3	**Fresh Garlic Cloves, minced**
1	**Small Yellow Onion, diced**
3 Cups	**Fresh Mushrooms**
1 Cups	**Marsala Wine**
2 Cups	**Shredded Mozzarella**

Fresh Basil for Garnish

Preheat oven to 350 degrees.

Trim the fat from each Chicken Breast. Cut each Chicken Breast in half by placing your hand flatly across the top. Cut horizontally from the thicker end to the thinner end.

Season the Flour with Oregano, Basil and Black Pepper. Put the Milk and Flour in separate wide bowls. Dip each Chicken Breast in milk and then dredge through the Bread Crumbs. Set aside.

In a heated large, heavy duty frying pan warm oil and half the butter over medium-high heat. Lay each Chicken Breast in the pan cooking approximately four (4) minutes each side. Add the

Minced Garlic after the first four (4) minutes. Place in large baking pan.

Heat remaining butter over medium/high heat. Once melted, add the Onions and Mushrooms cooking for two (2) minutes. Pour Marsala over Mushrooms, stirring to deglaze (scrape bits off the bottom) the pan.

Saute for another two (2) minutes. Pour mixture over Chicken.

Sprinkle Mozzarella Cheese over all the chicken. Bake, covered, for approximately fifteen (15) minutes. Remove foil and cook another five (5) minutes.

Place Chicken on plate, garnish with Basil.

Serve with Rice or Gluten Free Pasta.

Italian Meatballs

2 Lbs	**Ground Beef**
1 Lb	**Ground Pork**
1 C	**GFree Bread Crumbs**
	(Italian Seasoned)
½ C	**Onions, diced**
¼ C	**Grated Parmesan Cheese**
3 Cloves	**Fresh Garlic, minced**
2	**Eggs**
2 Tbs	**Oregano**
1 Tbs	**Basil**
1 Tbs	**Salt**
1 Tbs	**Pepper**
3 Tbs	**Olive Oil**
2 Tbs	**Butter**
1	**3oz Ice Cream Scoop**

Preheat oven to 400 degrees

In large bowl combine Beef and Pork by hand until it is mixed well. Add all the remaining ingredients and mix well. Scoop even portions of mixture using Ice Cream Scoop and place on non-stick cookie sheet ¼ inch apart. When the cookie sheet is full begin rolling each portion between your palms until a somewhat firm ball forms. Return to cookie sheet.

Heat a skillet and add the Olive Oil. When the Olive Oil is up to temperature, place Meatballs in the pan and saute. Add the Butter after turning the

Meatballs, spooning the Oil and Butter over the Meatballs for a flavorful crust.

Then place in the oven on a cookie sheet or in a stock pot of simmering Spaghetti Sauce to finish cooking
.

TIPS:

- For a less greasy alternative eliminate frying and instead bake covered for twenty (20) minutes. Remove foil and cook twenty (20) minutes more or until internal temperature is 165 degrees.

This is an easy dish for a busy school night. The recipe works with boneless or bone-in Pork Chops. The bone-in Chops will require a longer cook time. - DPS

Breaded Pork Chops

4	Pork Chops
½ Cup	All-Purpose GFree Flour
½ Cup	Milk
1 Cup	GF Bread Crumbs
2 tsp	Black Pepper
1 tsp	Oregano
1 tsp	Garlic Powder
1 tsp	Onion Powder
1 tsp	Salt

Preheat oven to 400 degrees.

Place three (3) medium size bowls on the counter.

Place the All-Purpose Gluten Free Flour in a medium size bowl. Add all the seasonings and blend together with a fork.

Pour the Milk in another medium size bowl.

Place the Gluten Free Bread Crumbs in a third (3rd) bowl.

Dredge the Pork Chop through the seasoned Flour making sure to coat completely.

Next dunk the Floured Pork Chop into the Milk.

Dredge through the seasoned Bread Crumbs.

Spread out on a baking sheet and cook thirty (30) minutes or until the Pork is 165 degrees.

Serve with Creamy Mashed Potatoes or steamed vegetables.

TIPS:

- My kids like to put the Bread Crumbs in a bag and shake the breading onto the Chops.

This is a family favorite for us. The homemade Barbecue Sauce and Potato Hamburger Buns are excellent combinations for a treat that always hits the spot! If you have a smoker then you don't need to use the slow-cooker method. Simply smoke for 6-8 hours at 195 degrees. - DPS

Pulled Pork Sliders

5-7 Lbs	**Boneless Pork Shoulder**
1	**Medium Onion**

Rub

¼ Cup	**Light Brown Sugar**
¼ Cup	**Paprika**
3 Tbs	**Fresh Black Pepper**
3 Tbs	**Salt**
2 Tbs	**Smoked Chipotle Pepper**
1 Tbs	**Garlic Powdered**
1 Tbs	**Onion Powder**
1 tsp	**Liquid Smoke**

Please see the recipes for Potato Hamburger Rolls and Barbecue Sauce.

Place all the Rub ingredients in a medium size bowl and stir until mixed well. Sprinkle the rub all over the Pork and begin rubbing it onto the meat with your fingers. Turn the meat and continue adding and rubbing until the Pork is completely covered.

Peel and Slice the Onion into thick rings. Lay half the Onion rings along the bottom of the slow-cooker. Pour the Chicken Stock over the rings. Put the pork on the Onions. Lay remaining Onion rings on top of the Pork. Set the timer for eight (8) hours or more.

Once the time is up press a fork into the Pork and gently pull. It should pull apart easily. If not, turn the cooker on it's shortest time setting, this will be it's highest heat and cook until the Pork pulls apart.

Pull all the Pork apart and keep it in the juices until needed.

Open the Potato Roll and using tongs place a heaping portion on the roll. Top with Homemade Barbecue Sauce.

Roast Beef

4 Lb	**Beef Sirloin Roast**
¼ Cup	**Virgin Olive Oil**
3	**Fresh Garlic Cloves**
1 Tbs	**Salt**
1 Tbs	**Ground Black Pepper**
1 Tbs	**Onion Powder**
1 tsp	**Paprika**
2 Tbs	**Dried Rosemary**

Allow the Roast to stand at room temperature at least one hour before cooking.

Preheat oven to 425 degrees.

In a small bowl add all the dry ingredients except the Dried Rosemary.

Rub oil over the Roast until completely covered. Pour dry ingredients over the top of the Roast and rub into the meat until completely covered.

Put Roast on a rack in a roasting pan. Sprinkle Roast with Dried Rosemary.

Place in oven, uncovered, for one (1) hour at 425 degrees. After one hour, turn off oven and keep the Roast in the oven for two (2) more hours.

Thirty (30) minutes before serving, turn oven on to 300 degrees. Cook for thirty (30) minutes and remove from the oven. Cut portions and serve at once.

TIPS:

- Keep the oven closed the entire three (3) hours the Roast is cooking.
- Letting the Roast sit for ten (10) minutes after removing from the oven will bring it to a Medium Rare finish.

Shrimp & Lobster Pasta

2	**Lobsters**
1 Lbs	**Shell-On Shrimp**
½ Lbs	**Scallops**
4	**Garlic Cloves**
1 Box	**Gluten Free Spaghetti**
½ Lbs	**Butter**
1 Cup	**Fresh Parsley**
2	**Lemons**
	(one whole, one sliced)

Bring a large pot ¾ full of water to a boil. Sprinkle a pinch of Salt in the water.

Add the Lobsters to the boiling water. Boil the Lobsters for a few minutes until the shell turns red and the tail is curled inward. Using tongs, pull the Lobster from the pot and set aside to drain. If you've bought Lobsters that are precooked, skip this step.

Add the Shrimp to the boiling water. Cook for only two (2) minutes. Using a slotted spoon pull the shrimp from the pot and put into a colander to drain & cool. Reduce the heat to low and simmer the water.

Peel the shells from the Shrimp, including the tail. Return the shells to the simmering water to create a Shellfish Broth. Run a sharp paring knife along the back and remove the dark vein. Set the Shrimp aside.

Crack the Lobster claws and tails to remove the meat. Return the claw and tail shells to the simmering water. Chop the Lobster meat into one (1) inch portions.

Peel and mince the Garlic.

In a second saucepan bring two (2) cups of water to a boil. Add three large ladles of the simmering Broth to this pan. **Be sure to keep the shells out.** Add the box of Gluten Free Spaghetti to the water/broth mixture and cook until Al Dente (approx 7 minutes). Drain & set aside.

In a large skillet melt half the Butter over medium-high heat. Add the Garlic and cook for two (2) minutes. Saute the Scallops for two (2) minutes each side. Add the Lobster and saute for another two (2) minutes. Add the Shrimp and stir.

Add the juice of one lemon to the seafood. Pour the Spaghetti into the skillet with the shellfish. Toss gently to incorporate. Add more Broth if needed.

Sprinkle with the Fresh Parsley and garnish with the sliced Lemon. Serve immediately.

This is a quick and simple dinner that the kids can help with. Our family prefers the sweetness of our homemade Teriyaki Sauce, but the more traditional recipe with Gluten Free Soy Sauce is included below. - DPS

Stir Fry Chicken & Veggies

4 lg	**Chicken Breasts (trimmed)**
2 Cups	**Rice cooked**
¼ Cups	**Vegetable Oil**
1 Cups	**GF Soy or Teriyaki Sauce**
1 Cups	**Snow Peas**
8	**Green Peppers**
4	**Yellow Onions**
1 Cups	**Mushrooms**
1 Cups	**Broccoli Florets**
4	**Cloves Garlic, minced**
1 can	**Water Chestnut**

Cut Chicken into one (1) inch cubes. Slice Green Peppers into one (1) inch strips. Slice Onions into one (1) inch strips. Chop Broccoli into one (1) inch pieces. Cut or slice Mushrooms into one (1) inch pieces.

Heat a large skillet or Wok on high heat. Add Oil and add Chicken, stirring until it turns white. Add Green Peppers and cook 2 minutes. Add Snow Peas and Onions. Continue cooking and stirring.

Add Garlic, Broccoli, Mushrooms and Water Chestnuts, cooking for 2 minutes. Pour Gluten Free

Soy Sauce over everything and continue stirring.
Lower the heat to keep warm.

Prepare Rice according to package directions. Place
Rice and Chicken on table and serve family-style.

TIPS:

- Don't precook the Broccoli. Let it cook in
  the hot pan with the other veggies.
- Add different colored peppers for flavor and
  colors.
- The "old fashion way" calls for dredging the
  Chicken in a batter of 3/4 cup of cornstarch
  with one (1) Cup of Sherry.

DESSERTS

Apple Crisp

10	**Medium size apples (Macintosh are best)**
¾ Cups	**Granulated Sugar**
1 Cups	**All Purpose GF flour**
1 Cups	**Light Brown Sugar**
1 Cups	**Rolled Oats (Gluten Free)**
1 tsp	**Baking Powder**
8 Tbs	**Very Cold Butter ,diced**
2 Tbs	**Cinnamon**
1 Tbs	**Nutmeg**
1 Tbs	**Shortening**

Core, peel and slice the Apples. Set aside. Grease large, glass brownie pan (9x13) with the shortening. Add Apples to pan and spread until they are evenly spaced. Sprinkle with Granulated Sugar. Dust with half Cinnamon.

In a separate bowl combine the Gluten Free All Purpose Flour, Light Brown Sugar, Rolled Oats, Nutmeg and remaining Cinnamon. Stir with a large fork until well blended.

Add a few pieces of the cold diced butter. Mix by hand squeezing the butter and dry mix until crumbly. Continue until all the butter is mixed into coarse crumbs. Spread over apples.

Bake uncovered one hour.

Chocolate Chip Cookies

2 Cups	White Rice Flour
¼ Cup	GF All Purpose Flour
¾ Cup	Sugar
¾ Cup	Brown Sugar
1 Cup	Butter softened
2	Eggs
1 tsp	Baking Soda
1 tsp	Vanilla Extract
1 tsp	Salt
2 tsp	Xanthum Gum
1 bag	Chocolate Chocolate Chips

Preheat oven to 375 degrees.

In a mixing bowl on medium speed, beat the Butter until creamy. Slowly add Eggs and Vanilla until mixed well.

In another bowl combine all dry ingredients stirring until well blended.

On a low speed, add dry ingredients slowly to Butter mixture. Add Chocolate Chips and continue mixing until combined.

Drop spoonfuls of cookie dough onto an ungreased cookie sheet. Bake eight (8) minutes or a bit longer until lightly browned.

Chocolate Peanut Butter Pie

Crust:

1 Cup	**GFree Graham Cracker Crumbs**
¼ Cup	**Brown Sugar**
¼ Cup	**Butter, melted**

Filling:

2 Cups	**Creamy Peanut Butter**
2 Cups	**Powdered Sugar**
16oz	**Cream Cheese, softened**
1½ Cups	**Heavy Cream**
2 Tbs	**Butter, melted**
2 tsp	**Vanilla Extract**

Topping:

1 Cup	**Semi-Sweet Chocolate**
3 Tbs	**Butter**

In medium bowl add Gluten Free Graham Cracker Crumbs and Brown Sugar. Add ¼ Butter (melted) and mix well. Press mixture in a large pie pan and chill for thirty (30) minutes.

In a mixing bowl add all the filling ingredients except the Heavy Cream. Using the paddle attachment, blend on medium speed. Slowly add the Heavy Cream. Increase speed to high until the mixture is whipped and light. Pour filling into pie crust shell. Place in refrigerator for six (6) hours until set.

Over a double-boiler melt three (3) tablespoons of Butter. Slowly add Chocolate Chips constantly stirring until well blended. If the Chocolate is sticking add two (2) tablespoons of Milk. When Chocolate topping is melted, pour over pie filling. Spread Chocolate topping until the top of the pie is covered. Return to refrigerator another hour for the Chocolate topping to set.

TIPS:

- Serve with whipped cream and shaved chocolate

Easy Milk Chocolate Truffles

2 Cups   **Milk Chocolate Chips**
1/3 Cup   **Heavy Cream**
6 Tbs   **Butter**

In a medium sauce pan heat Heavy Cream, but do not boil. Add the Butter and stir until melted. Slowly add Chocolate, constantly stirring until the Chocolate has melted and the mixture is smooth. Pour into a bowl and refrigerate for three (3) hours.

Using a small scoop or melon baller scoop mixture and drop on a plate. Roll the ball in your hands until smooth. Serve or store refrigerated until ready to use.

TIPS:

- Top the Truffles after rolling in your hands with coconut, peanuts, chocolate sprinkles or powdered sugar by pouring topping in a small bowl and roll the Truffles until covered.

Classic Apple Pie

1 Shell	3-2-1 GFree Pie Dough
4Cups	Apples, Peeled & Sliced
½ Cup	Light Brown Sugar
6 Tbs	Butter, cubed
1 tsp	Cinnamon
½ tsp	Nutmeg
1	Egg
½ Cup	All-Purpose GFree Flour
2 Pinch	Salt

Please see recipe for 3-2-1 Gluten Free Pie Dough in "Some Extra Stuff " section.

Preheat oven to 375 degrees. Grease a glass or ceramic pie pan.

Dust the work surface with a fair amount of the All-Purpose Gluten Free Flour. Cut pie dough in half. Roll out one half of the dough and place in the pie pan. Gently press the dough into the pan. Wet your fingers with cold water if necessary.

In a small bowl combine the Sugar, Cinnamon, Nutmeg and remaining All-Purpose Gluten Free Flour.

In a large bowl add the dry ingredients with the Apples to complete the filling, mixing gently. Pour the filling into the pie shell. Spread the cubes of Butter all over the top.

Roll out the other half of the dough large enough to cover the pie pan. In a small bowl scramble the Egg with about a Tablespoon of cold water and a pinch of Salt to create the Egg Wash. Brush the edges of the pie dough with the Egg Wash.

Lay the rolled out dough over the top of the pie pan. Trim the edges and crimp with your fingers to seal. Brush the remaining Egg Wash over the top of the pie. Sprinkle lightly with Salt. Slice a two inch hole in the top to vent while cooking.

Place the pie pan on a cookie sheet and bake for sixty (60) minutes or until the crust is golden brown.

TIPS:

- Slice the second half dough into strips and layer across the top of the filling for a lattice work finish.
- Serve warm with a scoop of Vanilla Ice Cream or Homemade Whipped Cream *(see "Some Extra Stuff" section)*.

Raspberry Squares

1 ¾ Cup	**Gluten Free Oats**
1 ½ Cup	**All-Purpose GFree Flour**
1 Cup	**Light Brown Sugar**
¾ Cup	**Butter**
1 tsp	**Xanthum Gum**
1 tsp	**Baking Soda**
½ tsp	**Salt**
10.5oz Can	**Raspberry Filling or Jam**

Preheat oven to 350 degrees.

In a large bowl add the Gluten Free Oats, Flour, Baking Soda, Salt, Brown Sugar and Xanthum Gum. Stir with a large spook or fork until well blended.

Melt Butter and pour into the bowl of dry ingredients. Combine mixture with your hands until it develops into moist crumbs.

Grease 8x8 or 9x9 square pan.

Reserve ¼ Cup and gently press remaining crumbs into the pan.

Spread Raspberry Filling over crumbs. Keep the filling away from the edges to prevent burning.

114

Drop the ¼ Cup of crumbs all over the top of the filling.

Bake for forty (40) minutes.

Let cool before cutting.

TIPS:

- If using store bought Jam, choose a seedless option.
- Greased foil can be used in the pan instead of greasing the pan itself
- Add miniature chocolate chips or slivers of Almonds to enhance the flavor.

Triple Chocolate Cupcakes

1 Cup	**All-Purpose GFree Flour**
1 Cup	**Granular Sugar**
½ Cup	**Baker's Chocolate Cocoa**
¼ Cup	**Vegetable Oil**
6 Tbs	**Butter**
3	**Eggs**
1 Tbs	**Vanilla Extract**
½ Cup	**Water**
1 Bag (11.5oz)	**Milk Chocolate Chips**

Preheat oven to 350 degrees.

Butter and Eggs should be taken out ahead of time to warm & soften.

In a medium size bowl pour Flour and Chocolate Cocoa. Stir and set aside.

In a small bowl, whisk the Eggs and set aside.

In a mixing bowl add Sugar, Butter, Vegetable Oil and Vanilla Extract. Beat on medium speed for two (2) minutes until smooth. Slowly add the Eggs until fully blended.

Gradually add the Flour and Chocolate Cocoa while beating on low speed. Slowly add water until batter comes together.

Add Chocolate Chips and blend on low speed for thirty (30) seconds.

Line muffin pan with cupcake papers. Scoop batter into each cup, about half-full.

Bake twenty (20) minutes or until toothpick is inserted and comes out clean. Let the cupcakes cool a few minutes before removing from the pan.

Frost with Homemade Chocolate Frosting.

TIPS:

- *If your cupcakes aren't rising or are collapsing, add small package of gelatin to the batter*
- *Substitute Peanut Butter Chips for the Milk Chocolate Chips.*
- *Add chocolate shavings or sprinkles on top of the frosting to finish.*

BREAKFAST

Easy Cinnamon Rolls

2 1/2 Cups	**GFree All Purpose Flour**
2 Tbs	**Baking Powder**
½ tsp	**Baking Soda**
½ tsp	**Salt**
1 tsp	**Xanthum Gum**
1 Tbs	**Active Dry Yeast**
¼ Cup	**Sugar**
1 ¼ Cups	**Milk**
1 Tbs	**Butter, melted**
1	**Egg**

Filling:

¼ Cup	**Butter, melted**
½ Cup	**Brown Sugar**
2 tsp	**Cinnamon**

Glaze:

¾ Cup	**Powdered Sugar**
¼ Cup	**Cream Cheese**
3 Tbs	**Butter, melted**
½ tsp	**Vanilla**

Preheat oven to 400 degrees

Warm the Milk & Butter in a small bowl. Add the Yeast and ¼ Cup of Sugar whisking together. Set aside to proof for ten (10) minutes.

In a mixing bowl add all the dry ingredients and stir together.

Add the Egg to the Yeast mixture. With mixer on a low speed add the Yeast mixture to the dry ingredients. Remove the dough from the bowl and knead it in your hands a few times.

Dust the work area with Flour and roll out the dough to a rectangular shape. Spread ¼ Cup of Butter just to the edges and sprinkle with Brown Sugar and Cinnamon.

Begin rolling from the side closest to you forward and away from you. Once you've created a long log cut in half. Then cut each half into four equal pieces. Continue cutting in half until each piece is 2-3 inches. Place in a greased pan and allow to rise for twenty (20) minutes. Bake for 20-25 minutes or until golden brown.

While the rolls are baking in a small bowl whisk the Powdered Sugar, Cream Cheese, Vanilla and remaining Butter until smooth. Drizzle the glaze over the rolls while they are still warm, but cooling. Serve warm.

Eggs Benedict for Two

4	**Fresh Eggs**
4	**Canadian Bacon slices**
2 Tbs	**White Vinegar**
2	**GFree English Muffins**
½ tsp	**Olive Oil or Butter**
1 Cup	**Hollandaise Sauce**
2	**Orange slices for garnish**
1 Tbs	**Chives, chopped for garnish**

Please see the Hollandaise Sauce recipe in the Sauce section

Prepare the Hollandaise Sauce first and set aside.

Crack each Egg into separate small bowls or tea cups.

To poach the Eggs, bring three (3) inches of water to almost a boil in a saucepan. Add two (2) tablespoons of White Vinegar. Stir the water with a spoon to create a swirling motion. Gently release one (1) Egg into the water. The Egg White should swirl right above the yolk and begin turning very white almost immediately. Add the second Egg in the same manner. Remove the pan from the heat.

After five (5) minutes very gently remove the Eggs from the water and set on a plate with a towel to dry.

Begin toasting the English Muffin if using a toaster oven. If pan-frying, wait until after the Bacon is browned.

Bring a small fry pan up to high heat. Add ½ teaspoon of Oil or Butter. Add the Canadian Bacon immediately and turn after one (1) minute. Continue frying until cooked (depending on the thickness, this could be another 1-2 minutes). Remove from the pan and set aside. If pan-frying the Muffin, add them now turning after two (2) minutes. After one (1) minute remove from pan and plate.

On a small plate center two (2) halves of the warm English Muffins. Top with one (1) slice each of the Canadian Bacon. Carefully place one (1) Egg on each of the Bacon slices. Ladle the Hollandaise Sauce over the Eggs. Sprinkle the Chives over the Sauce.

Garnish with the left over Chives, Parsley or an Orange slice.

Serve immediately.

Quiche Lorraine

12oz	**3-2-1 GFree Pie Dough**
	(see "Extra Stuff" section)
½ Lb	**Bacon, diced**
5	**Eggs**
2/3 Cup	**Gruyere or Swiss Cheese**
1 Cup	**Milk**
2/3 Cup	**Yellow Onion, chopped**
½ Cup	**Heavy Cream**

Preheat oven to 375 degrees

Prepare Gluten Free Pie Dough and place it in the pie pan. Score the pie crust either with a dough docker-wheel or by using a fork to perforate the pie crust.

Separate Yolk and Egg White of one Egg and scramble in a small bowl. Brush the pie shell with the Egg White.

In a small pan, fry the diced Bacon and Onion until the Bacon fat is rendered.

In another sauce pan, bring the Milk & Cream up to a temperature just below boiling. Set aside to cool.

In a bowl whisk the remaining Eggs. Add the slightly cooled Milk & Cream mixture. Stir in the Cheese along with the Bacon and onion and mix well. Pour into the waiting pie shell.

Bake for 40–45 minutes or until the top is golden brown.

TIPS:

- Substitute scallions for the sauteed Onion
- Add Mushrooms, Spinach or Tomato for a more hearty quiche
- Add breakfast sausage for a meatier quiche

Sweet Sunday Pancakes

1 Cup	**All-Purpose GFree Flour**
1 Tbs	**Granular Sugar**
½ Tbs	**Baking Powder**
½ tsp	**Salt**
1 tsp	**Vanilla Extract**
1	**Egg**
1	**Egg White**
2 Tbs	**Butter, melted**
¾ Cup	**Milk**

Preheat non-stick griddle.

In large bowl mix All-Purpose Gluten Free Flour, Sugar, Salt and Baking Powder with a whisk.

In a different bowl separate one (1) Egg discarding the yolk and keeping the Egg White. Add the second Egg. Pour Milk and melted Butter into the bowl and whisk vigorously. Add the Vanilla Extract and whisk together.

Add the wet mixture to the dry stirring until a smooth batter forms.

Pour mixture onto griddle in four (4) inch wide Pancakes. When bubbles begin to appear, especially along the sides they are ready to flip.

Once you've flipped the Pancakes they may puff up in size. Let this occur and flip a second time to their original position. The Pancakes should deflate. If not, gently press them down. If you press too soon you may cause the uncooked batter to leak on the griddle and your spatula.

Serve with additional Butter and _**original**_ Vermont Maple Syrup.

Waffles

1 Cup	**All-Purpose GFree Flour**
1 Tbs	**Granular Sugar**
1 Tbs	**Baking Powder**
½ tsp	**Baking Soda**
½ tsp	**Salt**
1 tsp	**Vanilla Extract**
2	**Eggs**
1	**Egg White**
2 Tbs	**Butter, melted**
¾ Cup	**Milk**

Preheat the Waffle Iron.

In large bowl mix All-Purpose Gluten Free Flour, Sugar, Salt, Baking Soda and Baking Powder with a whisk.

In a different bowl separate one (1) Egg discarding the yolk and keeping the Egg White. Add the other two (2) Eggs. Pour Milk and melted Butter into the bowl and whisk vigorously. Add the Vanilla Extract and whisk together.

Add the wet mixture to the dry stirring until a smooth batter forms.

Pour the batter onto the center of the Waffle Iron until it just reaches the outer ring. Close the lid and follow the instructions from the Waffle Iron.

Serve warm with Butter, Powdered Sugar and ***original*** Vermont Maple Syrup.

SOME EXTRA STUFF!!

Classic 3-2-1 Pie Dough

2 Cups	**All Purpose GFree Flour**
2/3 Cup	**Cold Water**
12 Tbs	**Cold Butter**

Cube the Butter by slicing the sticks in half length-wise. Then cut each half length-wise. Bring the stick back together and slice into small cubes approximately 1/4inches.

Combine the Flour with the Butter cubes by hand rubbing the mixture into tiny pieces. Add the Cold Water and continue mixing until a smooth dough forms. Refrigerate for about an hour to ninety (90) minutes.

Once the dough is cooled you can use immediately or freeze for later. Some recipes will require a pre-baked crust while others will call for the dough to be cooked together with the filling.

TIPS:

- The smaller the cube the quicker the mixing process.
- Use egg wash along the edges of the crust for securing the pie top and for brushing over the entire top to give it a golden brown finish.

Basic Chicken Stock

1	**Roasted Chicken Bones**
1 Cup	**Onion, chopped**
1 Cup	**Carrots, chopped**
1 Cup	**Celery, Chopped**
3	**Fresh Thyme Sprigs**
1 Tbs	**Parsley Flakes**
1 Tbs	**Salt**
1 Tbs	**Black Pepper**
3	**Bay Leaves**

Add all the ingredients to a large stock pot and fill with enough water to cover. Bring to a boil.

Reduce the heat to low and simmer for at least four (4) hours. For the first hour or so you will need to skim the surface of any fatty solids that collect.

After four (4) hours strain the ingredients from the liquid by pouring into another pot through a mesh strainer.

To use immediately, bring back to a boil and reduce by a quarter. If using later, transfer to a tightly sealed container and refrigerate until needed.

Tips:

If using raw Chicken

- Season a whole Chicken and Roast at 375 degrees until cooked. Usually thirty (30) minutes to the pound. Remove meat and set aside. Follow the instructions above. OR,
- De-bone the Chicken and place just the carcass in a roasting pan. Set the meat aside for another use. Add chopped Onion, Celery and Carrot. Season as above and cook at 375 degrees for about an hour or until the carcass is cooked. Remove from the oven and let cool slightly before adding to the stock pot. Then follow the instructions above. OR,
- Cut the roaster Chicken at every joint and carve the two breasts. Add 3 Tbs of Canola Oil to a stock pot and turn the heat to medium-high. Add the raw Chicken and bones to the stock pot and saute until cooked. Remove the Legs, Thighs, Wings and Breasts from the pot for another use. Follow the instructions above.

Gluten Free Garlic Croutons

1 Loaf	GFree White/Brown Bread
4 Tbs	Butter
1 Tbs	Basil
2 Tbs	Garlic Powder
1 Tbs	Parsley
1 Tbs	Paprika
1 Tbs	Salt
1 Tbs	Ground Black Pepper

Preheat oven to 375 degrees.

Butter both sides of each Gluten Free Bread slice. Dice or cube the Bread slices.

Melt remaining Butter in large frying pan and saute the cubes until browned on all sides. Place in a large bowl to cool.

In a small bowl mix all the spices. Sprinkle the mixed Spices over the sauteed Croutons and mix well. Or place Croutons and spices in a large bag and shake until Croutons are coated equally.

Lay out Croutons on a cookie sheet and bake in the oven until toasted. Set aside to cool.

Use once cooled or store in a container for later use.

Homemade Whipped Cream

1 Cup	**Heavy Cream**
4 Tbs	**Powdered Sugar**
	(aka Confectioner's Sugar)
½ tsp	**Vanilla Extract**

Using an electric hand mixer beat the Heavy Cream until it begins to thicken.

Gradually add the sugar and Vanilla Extract.

Continue mixing until it is light an airy.

Serve immediately.

TIPS:

- Other flavors can be added such as:
- Toasted Coconut, Maple Sugar, Chocolate Powder or Hazelnut.

Whipped Chocolate Frosting

2 ¼ Cups	**Confectioner's Sugar**
6 Tbs	**Bakers Cocoa Powder**
6 Tbs	**Butter**
3 Tbs	**Evaporated Milk**
2 Tbs	**Brewed Coffee, black**
1 tsp	**Vanilla Extract**
2 Pinch	**Salt**

In a large bowl cream the Butter by mixing on medium/high speed. Add the Evaporated Milk, Coffee and the Vanilla Extract.

In another bowl mix Sugar, Salt and Cocoa powder until well blended.

Add Sugar, Salt and Cocoa Powder and beat on medium speed another two(2) or three(3) minutes. Once the ingredients are blended and smooth, increase speed to high to create light, fluffy peaks.

Use immediately.

TIPS:

- Increase amount of Coffee or Sugar to adjust the taste
- Substitute Espresso or other strong coffee for a more robust flavor
- If cooking for kids who may not like the coffee flavor, substitute more Evaporated Milk for Coffee

134

Wonton Wrappers

1 Cup	**GFree All Purpose Flour**
1	**Egg**
1	**Egg White**
½ tsp	**Xanthum Gum**
¼ tsp	**Salt**
2 Tbs	**Water**

Keep some additional Flour handy to dust the work area and the rolling pin.

In a small bowl combine Egg, Egg White and Water. DO NOT scramble the Egg mixture.

In a larger bowl blend Flour, Xanthum Gum and Salt together. Add the Egg mixture slowly while stirring the Flour until the dough begins to form. It should be slightly sticky.

Sprinkle some of the additional Flour on your work area and the rolling pin. Divide the dough in half. Roll out one half of the dough until it is almost paper thin.

Cut the dough into even squares approximately 4x4 inches.

NOTES:

Acknowledgments

So there you have seventy or so recipes to get started. I've included many of the foods we enjoyed most as kids along with some new ideas we love! I hope you and your family enjoy them as well.

None of this would have been possible without the support and home recipe indexes my parents gave me so many years ago. Along with those index cards came "The Joy of Cooking." To me that book is easily the best reference book for any home cook. I still turn to mine often to brush up on old techniques or to confirm some of the food ideas swirling about in my head.

Over the years I've come across other cookbooks or recipes that we tried and have grown to love. I usually modify every recipe I come across to make it Gluten Free or to adjust to our kid's liking. You'll probably modify the recipes in this book too, so I left you "Notes" pages to do so.

I intend to give proper credit whenever possible. Unless specified below, most of the recipes in this collection come from our family index cards or are recipes we've received from friends.

"The Joy of Cooking" (1980 edition, Irma Rombauer & Marion Rombauer Becker): Crab Salad Won Ton, Sweet Potato Casserole, Chicken Cacciatore, Chocolate Truffles, Croutons, Whipped Chocolate Frosting, Won Ton Wrappers.

"Gluten Free Baking with the C.I.A." (2008 edition, Richard Coppedge Jr):
French Baguette, 3-2-1 Pie Dough, Naan -(my variation of his recipes)

"Italian Favorites" (2004 edition, Williams & Sonoma Kitchen Library):
Chicken Marsala, Bechamel Sauce, Hollandaise (my variation of their recipes)

Thank you to everyone who has shared ideas, insight, food, wine & most of all, their time. My sincerest apologies if I've forgotten anyone.

Kind Regards,

Daren

Please check out our videos on our YouTube Channel: gfreefoodtv

https://www.youtube.com/channel/UCPzEu29jYGA PZEhF9Bm0abw

Index

A

B

C

Cinnamon Rolls, 119-120
Cream (Whipped), 133
Croutons, 132
Cocktail Sauce, 22
Cocktail Sausages or Meatballs, 54-55
Coleslaw, 38

E
Eggs Benedict, 121-122

G
Grape Leaves (stuffed), 63-64
Green Beans, 71-72
Green Peppers, 80-81
Guacamole, 60

H
Hollandaise Sauce, 19
Hummus
       Classic, 61
       Mint, 62

M
Meatballs
       Italian, 94-95
       Cocktail, 54-55
Mushrooms (Stuffed), 65-66

N
Naan, 32-33